# LOW-C.

# RECIPES

*Soups*

## The Complete Guide With Simple and Yummy Low-Carb Recipes to Impress Your Friends And Family

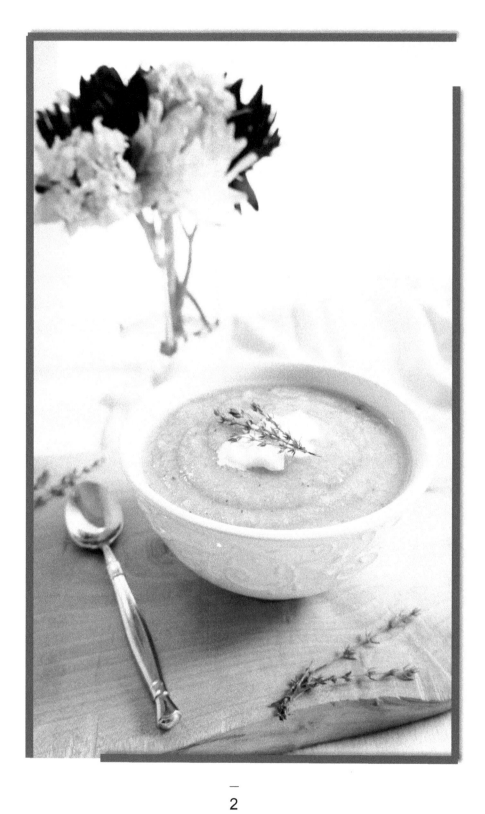

# Soups

Everybody loves soup.

Unfortunately, way too many people think of soup as something that comes out of a can or a packet, and the vast majority of packaged soups have added corn syrup or corn starch, plus, of course, things like rice, noodles, potatoes, beans, and other ingredients we simply can't have.

So make some soup yourself.

Most of these soups are quite simple to make, and many of them are filling, nutritious, one-dish meals.

Making a big batch (or even a double batch) of soup over the weekend is one of the greatest things you can do to save cooking time all week long.

If you want to make a soup as an appetizer or snack, choose one of the soups with lowest carb counts.

On the other hand, if you want a lunch or supper, keep an eye on the protein content, and figure that the vegetables in the soup will be all your carbs for that meal.

Note: You'll find that packaged broth generally comes in two sizes: I-quart cans and 14 Ih-ounce cans. Why this should be, I have no idea. But in any of these recipes, if you substitute two 14 Ih-ounce cans for 1 quart of broth, no harm will come to your soup, you'll just get slightly less volume. You can make up the difference with water, if you really want to, but I don't see why you'd bother.

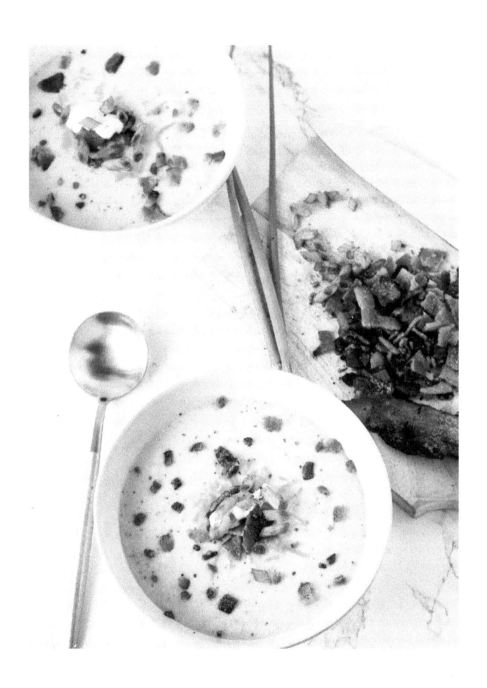

# *California Soup*

A quick and elegant first course.

1 large or 2 small, very ripe avocados, pitted, peeled,
and cut into chunks
1 quart chicken broth, heated

Put the avocados through the blender with the broth,
puree until very smooth, and serve.

Yield: 6 servings (as a first course), each with 3 grams
of carbohydrates and 1 gram
of fiber, for a total of 2 grams of usable carbs and 4
grams of protein.

~ If you like curry, you've got to try this: Melt a
tablespoon or so of butter
and add 1/2 teaspoon or so of curry powder. Cook for
just a minute, and
add the mixture to the blender with the broth and
avocados.

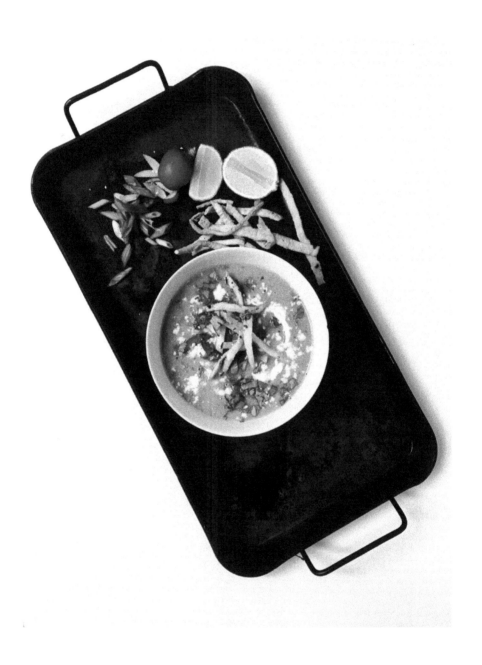

# *Artichoke Soup*

3 to 4 tablespoons butter
1 small onion, finely chopped
2 stalks celery, finely chopped
1 clove garlic, crushed
1 can (14 ounces) quartered artichoke hearts, drained
4 cups chicken stock
1/2 teaspoon guar or xanthan
1 cup half-and-half
Juice of 1/2 lemon
Salt or Vege-Sal
Pepper

1. In a heavy skillet, melt the butter and saute the onion, celery, and garlic over low to medium heat. Stir from time to time.
2. Drain the artichoke hearts, and trim off any tough bits of leaf that got left on. Put the artichoke hearts in a food processor with the S blade in position. Add 1/2 cup of the chicken stock and the guar gum, and process until the artichokes are a fine puree.
3. Scrape the artichoke mixture into a saucepan, add the remaining chicken stock, and set over medium-high heat to simmer.
4. When the onion and celery are soft, stir them into the artichoke mixture. When it comes to a simmer, whisk in the half-and-half. Bring it back to a simmer, squeeze in the lemon juice, and stir again. Salt and pepper to taste. You can serve this immediately, hot, or in summer you can serve it chilled.

Yield: 6 servings, each with 10 grams of carbohydrates and 3 grams of fiber, for a total of 7 grams of usable carbs and 4 grams of protein. (Note: Much of the carbohydrates in artichokes is inulin, which remains largely undigested, so this carb count is

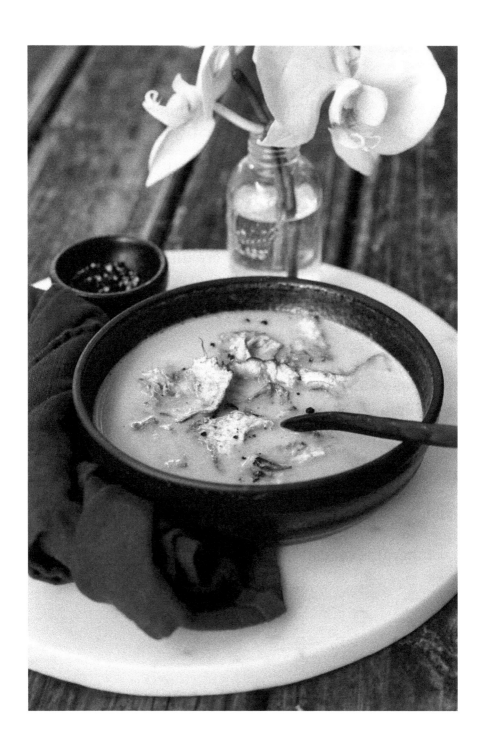

# *Olive Soup*

Olives are so good for you that you should be eating more of them! This makes a fine first course.

4 cups chicken stock
1/2 teaspoon guar or xanthan
1 cup minced black olives (you can buy cans of
minced black olives)
1 cup heavy cream
1/4 cup dry sherry
Salt or Vege-Sal
Pepper

1. Put 1/2 cup of the chicken stock in the blender with the guar gum, and blend for a few seconds. Pour into a saucepan, and add the rest of the stock and the olives.
2. Heat until simmering, then whisk in the cream. Bring back to a simmer, stir in the sherry, and salt and pepper to taste.

Yield: 6 servings, each with 3 grams of carbohydrates and 1 gram of fiber, for a total of 2 grams of usable carbs and 2 grams of protein.

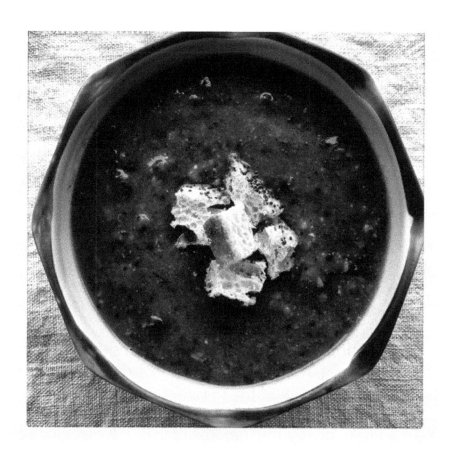

# Turkey Meatball Soup

This makes a light, quick, and tasty supper all by itself.

1/2 pound ground turkey
1 1/2 tablespoons oat bran
2 tablespoons minced fresh parsley
1/2 teaspoon salt or Vege-Sal
1/2 teaspoon poultry seasoning
1/8 teaspoon pepper
1 tablespoon olive oil
1/2 CU P grated ca rrot
2 cups diced zucchini
1 tablespoon minced onion
1 clove garlic, crushed
1 quart chicken broth
1 teaspoon dried oregano
2 eggs, beaten
1/4 cup grated Parmesan cheese

1. In a mixing bowl, combine the ground turkey with the oat bran, parsley, 1/2 teaspoon salt or Vege-Sal, poultry seasoning, and pepper. Mix well, and form into balls the size of marbles or so. Set aside.
2. In a large, heavy-bottomed saucepan, heat the olive oil over a medium-high burner.
Add the carrot, and let it saute for 2 to 3 minutes. Then add the zucchini, onion, and garlic, and saute the vegetables for another 5 to 7 minutes.
3. Add the chicken broth and oregano, and bring the soup to a simmer for 15 minutes.

Drop the turkey meatballs into the soup one by one, and let it simmer for another 10 to 15 minutes.

Taste the soup at this point, and add more salt and pepper to taste, if
desi red.

4. Just before you're ready to serve the soup, stir it slowly with a fork as you pour the
beaten eggs in quite slowly. Simmer another minute, and ladle into bowls. Top each serving with 1 tablespoon of Parmesan, and serve.

Yield: 4 servings, each with 7 grams of carbohydrates and 2 grams of fiber, for a
total of 5 grams usable carbs and 21 grams of protein.

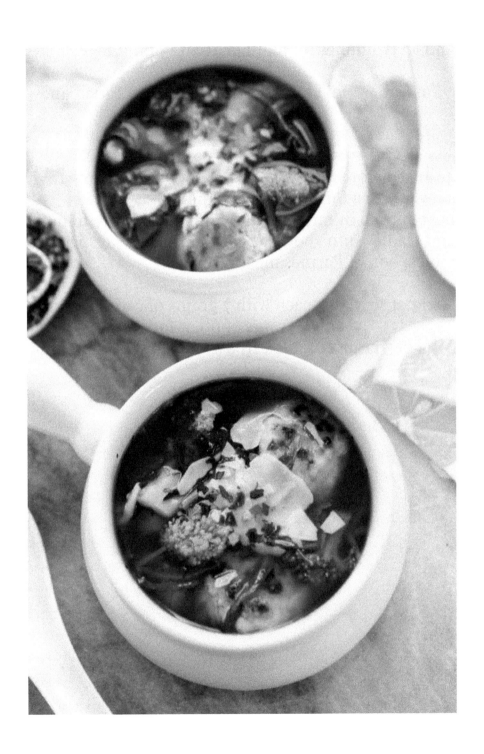

# Kim's Week-After-Thanksgiving Soup

This is what my sister did with the carcass from her Thanksgiving turkey. Our mother always made turkey and rice soup, but we lowcarbers needed a new tradition, and here it is.

1 turkey carcass
1 tablespoon salt
2 tablespoons vinegar
5 small turnips, cut into largish cubes
4 ribs celery, cut into 1/2-inch lengths
1/2 pound mushrooms, sliced
1 large onion, chopped
2 zucchini, each about 6 inches long, diced into small chunks
2 cups frozen, cut green beans
1 chicken bouillon cube or 1 teaspoon chicken bouillon crystals
2 tablespoons dried basil
Salt and pepper

1. In a large pot, break up the turkey carcass, leaving bits of meat clinging to it. Cover it with water, add the salt and vinegar, and simmer on low until the water is reduced to about 4 quarts. Let cool.
2. Pour the whole thing through a strainer, and return the broth to the pot. Pick the meat off the turkey bones. Discard the bones, cut up the meat, and return it to the pot.

3. Add the turnips, celery, mushrooms, onion, zucchini, beans, bouillon, and basil, and simmer until the vegetables are soft. Salt and pepper to taste, and serve.

Yield: 12 servings, each with 12 grams of
carbohydrates and 4 grams of fiber, for a
total of 8 grams of usable carbs. Your protein count
will depend on how much meat
was left on your turkey carcass, but assuming 2 cups
of diced turkey total, you'll get
15 grams of protein per serving.

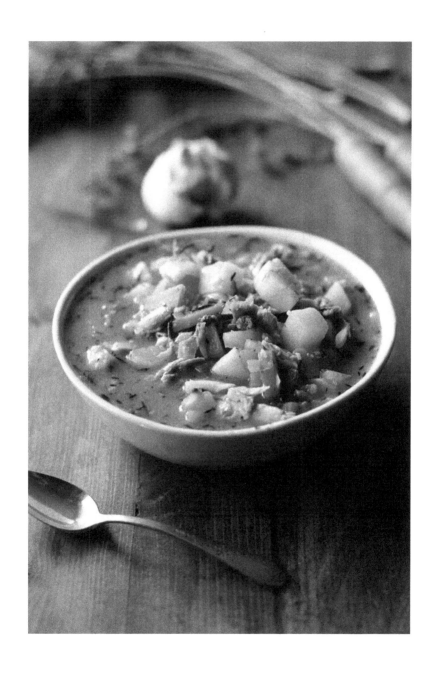

# Portuguese Soup

If this were really authentic, it would have potatoes in it. But this decarbed version is delicious, and it's a full meal in a bowl. Read the labels on the smoked sausage carefully-they range from 1 gram of carb per serving up to 5.

1/3 cup olive oil
3/4 cup chopped onion
3 cloves garlic, crushed
2 cups diced turnip
2 cups diced cauliflower
1 pound kale
1 1/2 pounds smoked sausage
1 can (14 1/2 ounces) diced tomatoes
2 quarts chicken broth
1/4 teaspoon Tabasco
Salt and pepper

1. Put 1/4 cup of the olive oil in a large soup pot, and saute the onion, garlic, turnip, and cauliflower over medium heat.
2. While that's cooking, chop the kale into bite-size pieces, and add it to the pot, as well. (You may need to cram it in at first, but don't worry-it cooks down quite a bit.) Let the vegetables saute for another 10 minutes or so, stirring to turn the whole thing over every once and a while.
3. Slice the smoked sausage lengthwise into quarters, then crosswise into 1/2-inch pieces. Heat the

remaining 2 tablespoons of oil in a heavy skillet over medium heat, and brown the smoked sausage a little.
4. Add the browned sausage, tomatoes, and 7 1/2 cups of the chicken broth to the kettle, and use the last 1/2 cup of broth to rinse the tasty browned bits out of the frying pan, and add that, too. Bring to a simmer and cook until the vegetables are soft (30 to 45 minutes). Stir in the Tabasco and salt and pepper to taste, and serve.

Yield: 10 servings, each with 13 grams of carbohydrates and 2 grams of fiber, for a total of 11 grams of usable carbs and 23 grams of protein.

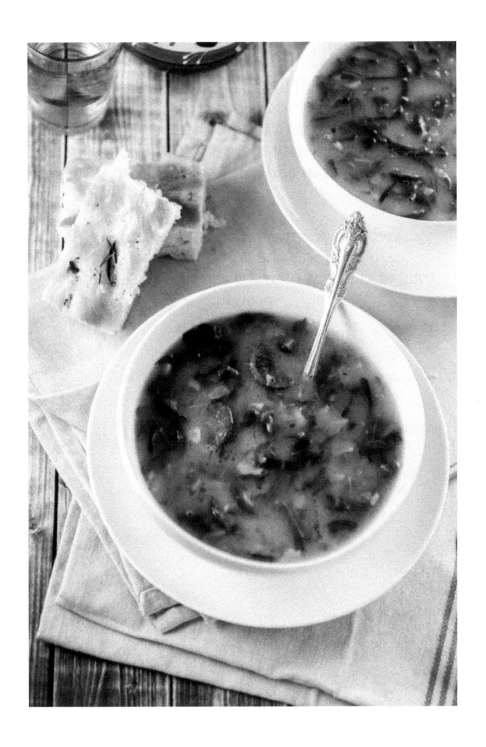

# *Corner-Filling Consomme*

2 tablespoons butter
4 ounces sliced mushrooms
1 small onion, sliced paper-thin
1 quart beef broth
2 tablespoons dry sherry
1/4 teaspoon pepper

Melt the butter in a skillet, and saute the mushrooms and onions in the butter until they're limp. Add the beef broth, sherry, and pepper. Let it simmer for 5 minutes or so, just to blend the flavors a bit, and serve.

Yield: 6 appetizer-size servings, each with 5 grams of carbohydrates and 1 gram of
fiber, for a total of 4 grams of usable carbs and 8 grams of protein.

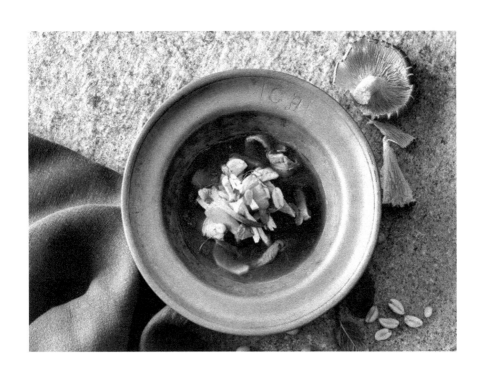

# *Crock-Pot Tomato Soup*

Delicious tomato soup from Splendid Low Carbing, by Jennifer Eloff of sweety.com. So easy!

2 1/2 cups V8 or other mixed vegetable juice
2 1/2 cups boiling water
8 ounces canned tomato sauce
1 small onion, thinly sliced
1 bay leaf
3 tablespoons Splenda
1 tablespoon beef bouillon granules or liquid beef-broth concentrate
1/8 teaspoon pepper
1/4 teaspoon dried basil
Combine all ingredients in a slow cooker and stir. Cover and cook on Low for
4 hours. Strain and serve.

Yield: 6 servings, each with 10 grams of carbohydrates and 2 grams of fiber, for a total or 8 grams of usable carbs and 2 grams of protein.

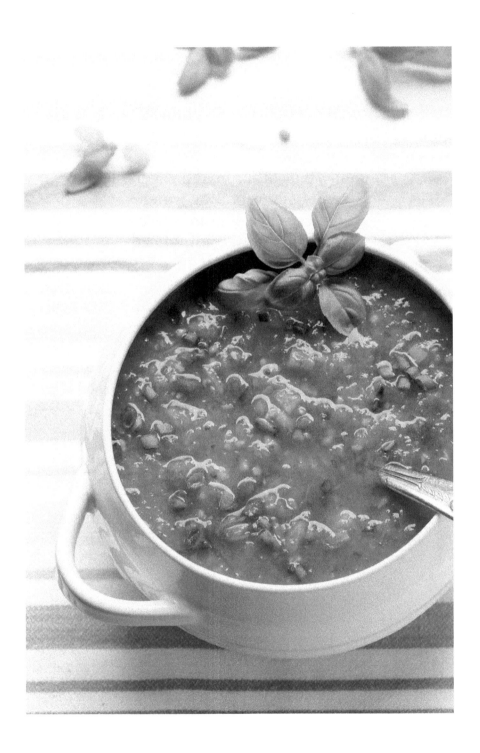

# *Mulligatawny*

This is a curried soup that came out of the British Colonial times in India. It's also wonderful made with broth made from a turkey carcass, or, for that matter, from the remains of a leg of lamb.

2 quarts chicken broth
2 cups or more diced cooked chicken or diced boneless, skinless chicken breast
3 tablespoons butter
1 clove garlic, crushed
1 medium onion, chopped
1 small carrot, shredded
2 ribs celery, diced
2 teaspoons to 1 1/2 heaping tablespoons curry powder
(I like it with lots of curry!)
1 bay leaf
1/2 tart apple, chopped fine
1 to 2 teaspoons salt or Vege-Sal
1/2 teaspoon pepper
1/2 teaspoon dried thyme
Rind of 1 fresh lemon, grated, or 1/2 to 1 teaspoon dried
1 cup heavy cream

1. Put the broth and diced chicken in a large stockpot, and set the stockpot over low heat.
2. Melt the butter in a heavy skillet, and add the onion, garlic, carrot, celery, and curry powder. Saute until the vegetables are limp, and add them to the stockpot.

3. Add the bay leaf, apple, salt, pepper, thyme, and lemon to the pot, and simmer for 1/2 hour. Just before serving, stir in the cream.

Yield: 6 servings, each with 8 grams of carbohydrates and 2 grams of fiber, for a
total of 6 grams of usable (arbs and 18 grams of protein.

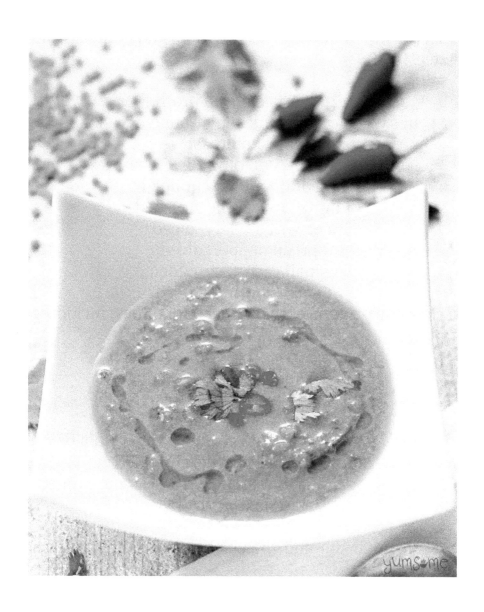

# *Sopa Azteca*

That's soup made by Aztecs, not soup made from Aztecs!

3 quarts chicken broth
2 cups diced cooked chicken or boneless, skinless chicken breast
1/4 cup olive oil
1 medium onion, chopped
4 or 5 cloves garlic, crushed
2 or 3 ribs celery, diced
1 green pepper, diced
1 small carrot, shredded
1 small zucchini, diced
2 cans (14 1/2 ounces each) diced tomatoes, including juice
1 package frozen chopped spinach
2 tablespoons dried oregano
2 tablespoons dried basil
2 teaspoons pepper
At least 8 ounces Mexican Queso Quesadilla or Monterey Jack cheese, shredded
Chipotle peppers in adobo sauce (these come canned)
5 ripe Haas avocados

1. Heat the broth and the chicken in a large pot over low heat.
2. Heat the olive oil in a skillet over medium heat, and saute the onion, garlic, celery, pepper, carrot, and zucchini together until they're limp. Stir the oregano, basil and pepper into thevegetables and sautee for

another minute and add them to the soup, along with the tomatoes and spinach. Let the whole thing simmer for 1/2 to 1 hour, to let the flavors blend.

3. When you're ready to serve the Sopa Azteca, put at least 1/4 to 1/2 cup of cheese (more won't hurt) in the bottom of each bowl, and anywhere from 1 to 3 chipotles, depending on how spicy you like your food. (If you don't like spicy food at all, leave the chipotles out entirely.) Ladle the hot soup over the cheese and peppers.

4. Use a spoon to scoop chunks of 1/2 ripe avocado onto the top of each bowl of soup.

Yield: 10 servings. Each serving of soup alone has 21 grams of carbohydrates and
6 grams of fiber, for a total of 15 grams of usable carbs and 25 grams of protein.
1/2 cup of shredded cheese adds only a gram or so of carbohydrates and 14 grams
of protein. Each chipotle pepper adds no more than 1 gram or so of carbs, and
1/2 a Haas avocado has about 6 grams of carbohydrates and 2.5 grams of fiber,
for a total of 3.5 grams of usable carbs per serving.

~ The totals on this soup may sound like a lot when you add them all up, but
don't forget that this is a whole meal in a bowl: meat, vegetables, melted
cheese, and lovely ripe avocado in each bite! You don't need to serve
another thing with it, although if you could serve tortillas or quesadillas

———

for the carb-eaters in the crowd.

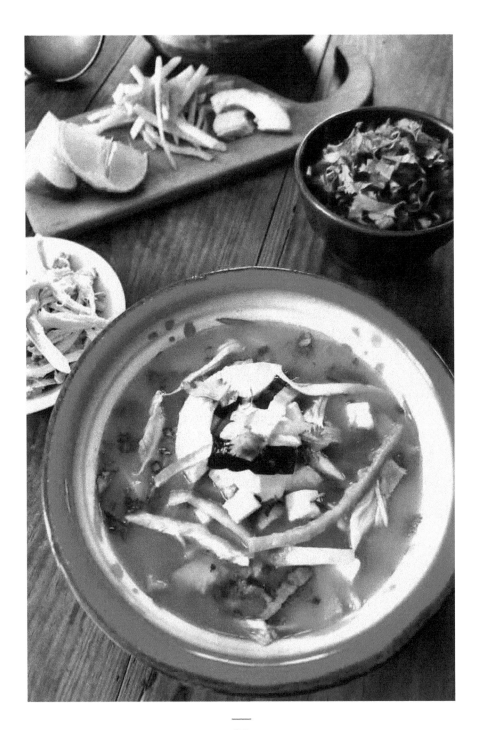

# *Hot-and-Sour Soup*

Really authentic Hot-and-Sour Soup uses Chinese mushrooms, but this is mighty good with any variety-especially when you have a cold!

2 quarts chicken broth
1 piece of fresh ginger about the size of a walnut, peeled and thinly sliced
1/2 pound lean pork (I use boneless loin.)
3 tablespoons soy sauce
1 to 1 1/2 teaspoons pepper
1/2 cup white vinegar
2 cans (6 1/2 ounces each) mushrooms
1 cake (about 10 ounces) firm tofu
1 can (8 ounces) bamboo shoots
5 eggs

1. Put the broth in a kettle and set it over medium heat. Add the ginger to the broth and let it simmer for a few minutes.
2. While the broth simmers, slice the pork into small cubes or strips. (I like strips.) Stir the soy sauce, pork, pepper, vinegar, and mushrooms (you don't need to drain them) into the broth. Let it simmer for 10 minutes or so, until the pork is done through.
3. Cut the tofu into small cubes. If you like, you can also cut the canned bamboo shoots into thinner strips. (I like them better that way, but sometimes I don't feel like doing the extra work.) Stir the tofu and bamboo shoots into the soup, and let it simmer another few minutes. Taste the soup; it won't be very hot-spicy-hot,

that is, not temperature-hot-so if you like it hotter, add more pepper and some hot sauce. If you like, you can also add a little extra vinegar.

4. Beat the eggs in a bowl, and then pour them in a thin stream over the surface of the soup. Stir them in, and you'll get a billion little shreds of cooked egg in your soup. Who needs noodles?

This is good served with a few finely sliced scallions on top (include some of
the green part) and a few drops of toasted sesame oil. Since I like my soup
hotter than my husband does, I use hot toasted sesame oil, rather than putting
hot sauce in the whole batch.

Yield: 6 servings, each with 10 grams of carbohydrates and 2 grams of fiber, for a total of 8 grams of usable carbs and 25 grams of protein.

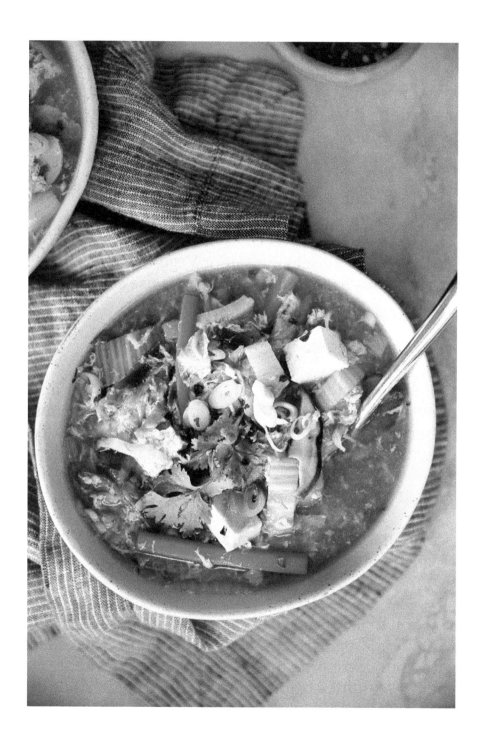

# *Peanut Soup*

If you miss split pea or bean soup, try this. Try it even if you don't miss other soups-you may find you have a new favorite.

3 tablespoons butter
2 or 3 ribs celery, finely chopped
1 medium onion, finely chopped
2 quarts chicken broth
1/2 teaspoon salt or Vege-Sal
1 1/4 cups natural peanut butter (I use smooth.)
1 teaspoon guar gum (optional)
2 cups half-and-half or heavy cream
Salted peanuts, chopped

1. Melt the butter in a skillet, and saute the celery and onion in the butter. Add the broth, salt, and peanut butter, and stir. Cover and simmer on the lowest temperature for at least 1 hour, stirring now and then.

~ If your slow cooker will hold this quantity of ingredients (mine will), it's ideal for cooking this soup. Set it on High, cover it, and let it go for 2 to 3 hours.

2. If you're using guar gum (it makes the soup thicker without adding carbs; most peanut soup is thickened with flour), scoop 1 cup of the soup out of the kettle about 15 minutes before you want to serve it. Add the guar gum to this cup, run the mixture through the

blender for a few seconds, and whisk it back into the soup.

3. Stir in the half-and-half, and simmer for another 15 minutes. Garnish with the peanuts.

Yield: 5 servings, The carb count will depend on what brand of natural peanut
butter you use (they have varying amounts of fiber) and whether you use half-andhalf
or heavy cream. Figure each serving has about 19 grams of carbohydrates and
3 grams of fiber, for a total of 16 grams of usable carbs and 29 grams of protein.

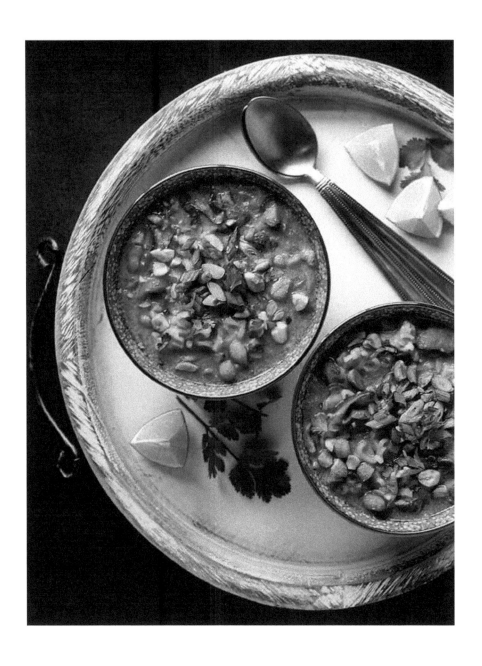

# *Spring Chicken Soup*

This soup is a great way to use up leftovers-just substitute 1 cup of leftover chicken for the chicken breast called listed with the ingredients.

6 cups chicken broth
1 can (6 1/2 ounces) mushrooms
1 can (6 1/2 ounces) cut asparagus
1 boneless, skinless chicken breast, diced into small cubes
1/4 cup dry sherry
1 tablespoon soy sauce
Pepper
Sliced scallions

Combine the broth, mushrooms, asparagus, chicken, sherry, and soy sauce in a pot, and heat. If you're using raw chicken, let it cook for 5 to 10 minutes (that's all it should take to cook small cubes of chicken through). Add pepper to taste, and serve
with a scattering of scallions on top.

If you're feeling ambitious, there's no reason you couldn't make this with
fresh mushrooms and fresh asparagus; you'll just have to simmer it a little
longer. As it is, though, this soup is practically instantaneous!

Yield: 4 servings. Depending on the broth you use, this should have no more than

---

about 17 grams of usable carbs in the whole pot, plus about 0.5 gram for the little bit of scallion you put on top of each bowl. Figure each serving has 6 grams of carbohydrates and 2 grams of fiber, for a total of 4 grams of usable carbs and 23 grams of protein.

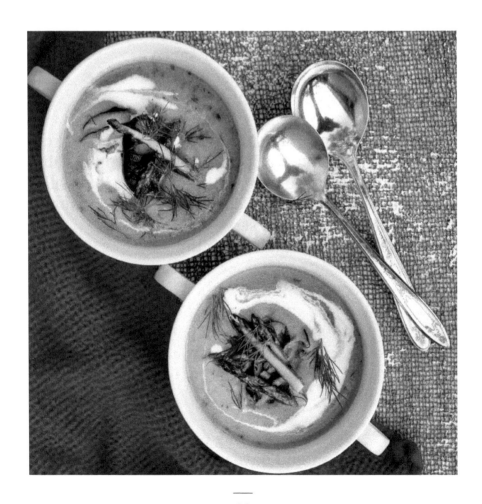

# Judie's Chicken "Noodle" Soup

Judie Edwards created this when she was craving chicken noodle soup, and it's a cinch to make.

2 cups chicken broth
1 can Chinese vegetables, drained
Simply combine, heat, and serve.

Yield: 1 serving, with 7 grams of carbohydrates and 2.5 grams of fiber, for a total of
4.5 grams of usable carbs and 7 grams of protein.

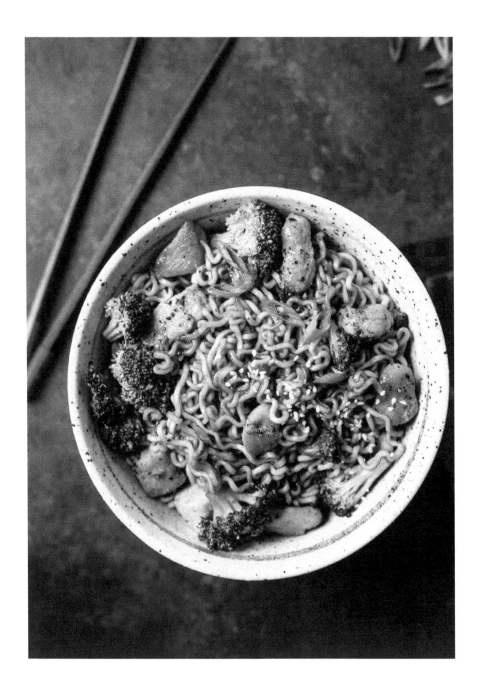

# *Easy Tomato-Beef Soup*

1/4 to 11/2 pound ground beef
2 cans (14 1/2 ounces each) beef broth
1 can (14 1/2 ounces) diced tomatoes

In a skillet, brown the ground beef. Pour off the grease, and add the broth and tomatoes. Heat through , and serve.

Yield: 4 servings, each with 9 grams of carbohydrates,
a trace of fiber, and
19 grams of protein.

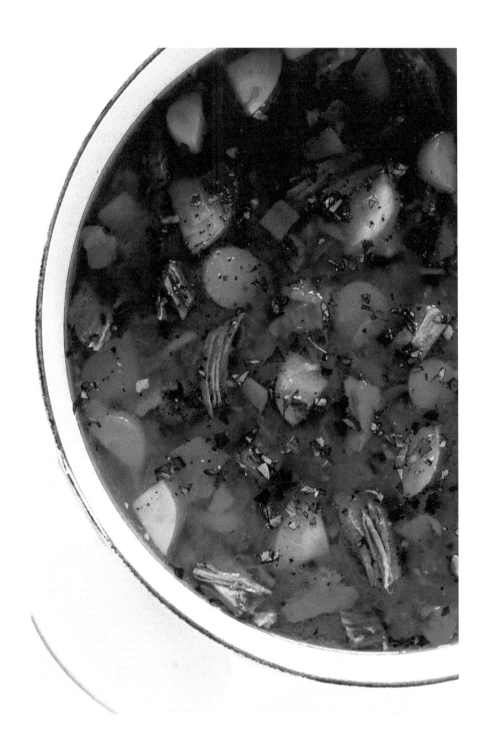

# *Italian Tuna Soup*

Okay, it's not authentically Italian, but it's a lot like minestrone. It's easy, too.

1 quart chicken broth
1 can (14 1/2 ounces) diced tomatoes
1 can (14 1/2 ounces) Italian green beans or 1 package (10 ounces) frozen
Italian green beans
1/2 cup frozen broccoli cuts
1/2 cup frozen cauliflower cuts
1 cup thinly sliced zucchini, frozen or fresh
3 tablespoons tomato paste
1 teaspoon Italian seasoning
2 cans (6 ounces each) tuna
Tabasco

Combine the broth, tomatoes, beans, broccoli, cauliflower, zucchini, tomato paste, seasoning, and tuna. Add a few drops of Tabasco (more if you like it hotter, less if you just want a little zip), and simmer until the vegetables are tender.

Yield: 5 servings, each with 14 grams of carbohydrates and 3 grams of fiber, for a total of 11 grams of usable carbs and 23 grams of protein.

~ Check the frozen foods section of your supermarket for mixed bags of broccoli

and cauliflower, and substitute 1 cup of the mix for the separate cauliflower
and broccoli. That way, you'll only have one partially eaten bag of
veggies in the freezer to use up, rather than two.

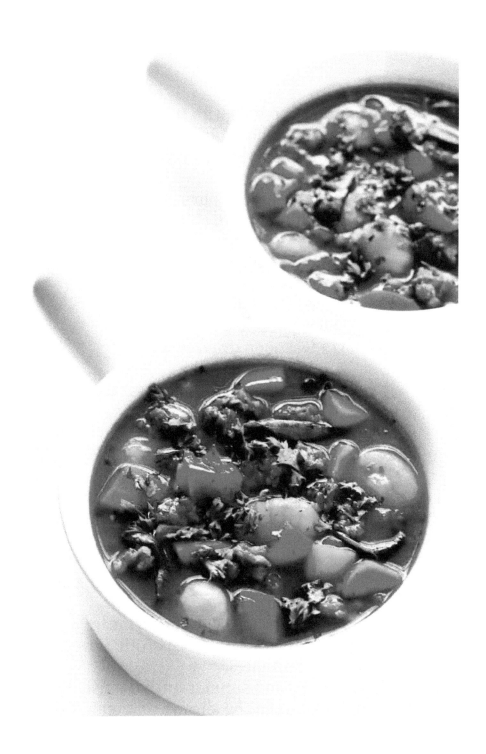

# Zesty Seafood Soup

Marilee Wellersdick came up with this. Just make sure you use real crab, not the high-carb fake crab that's widely available these days, when you make this soup.

2 tablespoons olive oil
1 medium onion, chopped
2 cloves garlic, minced
1 cup chopped celery
2 tablespoons fresh or dried parsley, chopped
1 teaspoon dried basil
1/2 teaspoon dried rosemary
1/2 teaspoon dried thyme
Dash of cayenne
3 cans (8 ounces each) tomato sauce
8 ounces clam juice
1 can (14 1/2 ounces) chicken broth
1 pound firm fish (such as cod, halibut, or snapper),
cut into 1-inch cubes
4 1/2 ounces small canned, fresh, or frozen shrimp
1 can (8 ounces) crabmeat, or 1 fresh crab
Salt

1. Heat the oil in a Dutch oven. Add the onion, garlic, and celery, and saute until the onion is limp.
2. Stir in the parsley, basil, rosemary, thyme, cayenne, tomato sauce, clam juice and chicken broth. Cover and simmer for about 10 minutes.
3. Add the fish; cover and simmer until the fish flakes (about 7 minutes). Stir in the shrimp and crab. Cover

and cook for a few minutes, until everything is thoroughly heated. Salt to taste.

Yield: About 8 servings, each with 12 grams of carbohydrates and 2 grams of fiber,
for a total of 10 grams of usable carbs and 12 grams of protein.

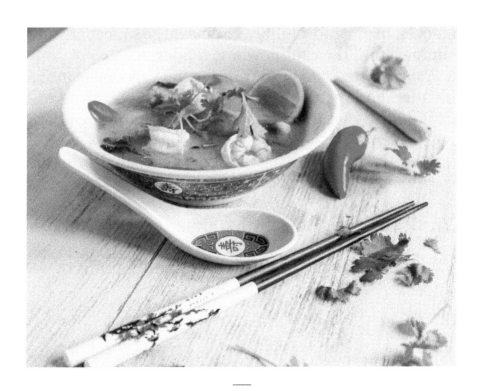

# *Cream of Cauliflower*

You'll be surprised by how much this tastes like Cream of Potato!

3 tablespoons butter
3/4 cup diced onion
3/4 cup diced celery
1 quart chicken broth
1 package (10 ounces) frozen cauliflower
1/2 teaspoon guar or xanthan (optional)
1/2 cup heavy cream
Salt and pepper

1. Melt the butter over low heat, and saute the onion and celery in it until they're limp. Combine with the chicken broth and cauliflower in a large saucepan, and simmer until the cauliflower is tender.
2. Use a slotted spoon to transfer the vegetables into a blender, and then pour in as much of the broth as will fit. Add the guar or xanthan (if using), and puree the i ngred ients.
3. Pour the mixture back into the saucepan. Stir in the cream, and salt and pepper to taste.

Yield: 4 servings, each with 9 grams of carbohydrates and 3 grams of fiber, for a
total of 6 grams of usable carbs and 7 grams of protein.

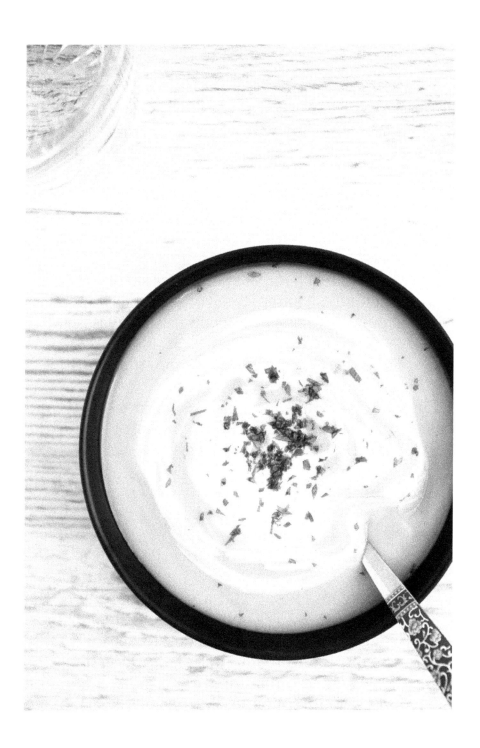

# Skydancer's Zucchini Soup

Jo Pagliassotti, an artist who works under the name Skydancer, came up with this savory and versatile soup.

4 cups chopped zucchini, cut into chunks
2 cups chopped Spanish onion
4 cups chicken stock, homemade or canned (if homemade, salt to taste)
1 to 2 teaspoons dry summer savory
or 1/4 cup fresh summer savory leaves, chopped
1 tablespoon dry basil or 1/2 cup fresh leaves, lightly packed
8 ounces cream cheese, at room temperature

1. Place the zucchini, onion, stock, summer savory, and basil into a pan. Cook over low heat until the vegetables are soft (30 minutes minimum).

It won't hurt this soup a bit if you turn the burner to low, cover the pan,
and forget it for a couple of hours. You want it to be squashy (pun intended!).

2. Put the cream cheese and a small quantity of the cooked mixture into a blender, and blend until smooth. (Add more liquid if needed to get the cheese smooth.) Pour that into another pan. Add more of the cooked squash and onion mixture to the blender, and blend until smooth (or as smooth as you like it). Blend

the rest of the cooked mixture, pouring each blended batch into the soup and cheese mixture as you go.

3. Once everything is pureed, stir it well to mix in the initial cheese and zucchini blend, and rewarm over low heat if necessary.

Yield: 9 servings, each with 6 grams of carbohydrates and 2 grams of fiber, for a total
of 4 grams of usable carbs and 3 grams of protein. Try making this with a mixture of yellow squash and zucchini, but note that yellow
squash has more carbs than zucchini. You can also use green onion or leeks instead
of the Spanish onion. Keep in mind that 2 cups of green onion will give you 9.6
grams of carbs instead of 22 and 2 cups of leeks will give you 61.6 grams of carbs
(why are they so high?) instead of 22.
Want even more variety and some more protein along with it? Leftover flaked
salmon and chunks of cold leftover chicken are both great in this. You can garnish
the soup with some sliced green onions or shallots, and that's also wonderful. This
soup lends itself to many variations-be creative. Oh, and it freezes well! The
cream cheese seems to hold up to this just fine.

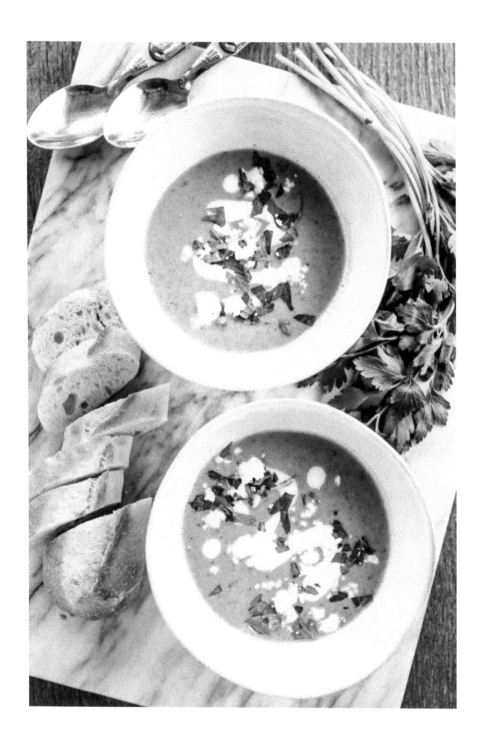

# Jodee's Zucchini Soup

Here's another take on zucchini soup, from reader Jodee Rushton. She says this is satisfying as a quick between-meals snack, not to mention versatile: "In the summer, pour it into a mug and drink it cold. In the winter, you might microwave it."

1/4 cup butter
1 medium onion, chopped
1 1/2 pounds zucchini, washed and sliced
28 ounces chicken broth
1/8 teaspoon salt
1/8 teaspoon pepper
1/2 teaspoon ground nutmeg
1/2 cup half-and-half

1. Melt the butter and saute the onion in it until golden. Add the zucchini and saute over medium-high heat until limp (10 to 15 minutes).
2. Add the chicken broth, salt, pepper, and nutmeg. Simmer for 15 minutes, add the half-and-half, and let the mixture cool.
3. Puree the broth mixture in a blender. (Do this in batches, if necessary.) Refrigerate for a minimum of 4 hours, to allow the flavors to blend. Serve hot or cold.

Yield: 8 servings, each with 5 grams of carbohydrates and 1 gram of fiber, for a total of 4 grams of usable carbs and 2 grams of protein.

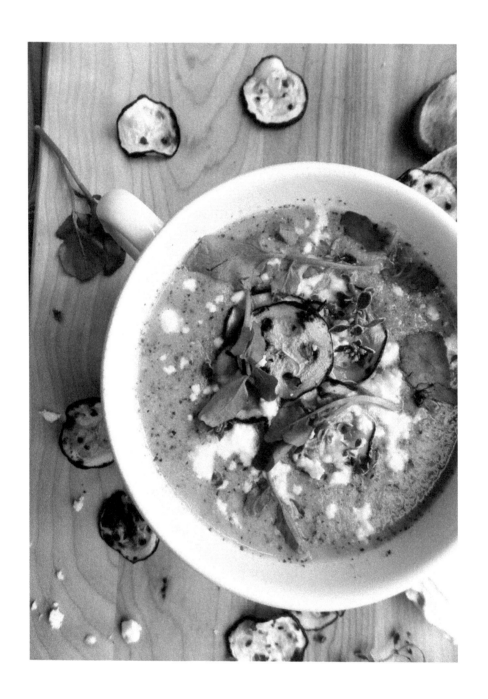

# Jamaican Pepperpot Soup

Unbelievably hearty, almost like a stew, and very tasty!

1/2 pound bacon, diced
2 pounds boneless beef round or chuck, cut into 1-inch cubes
1 large onion, chopped
4 cups water
1 cup canned beef broth
2 packages (10 ounces each) frozen chopped spinach
1/2 teaspoon dried thyme
1 green pepper, diced
1 can (14 1/2 ounces) sliced tomatoes
1 bay leaf
2 teaspoons salt
1/2 teaspoon pepper
1 teaspoon hot sauce (or to taste)
1 package (10 ounces) frozen sliced okra, thawed
3 tablespoons butter
1/2 cup heavy cream
Paprika

1. Place the bacon, beef cubes, onion, water, and beef broth in a large, heavy soup pot. Bring to a boil, turn the burner to low, and let the mixture simmer for 1 hour.
2. Add the spinach, thyme, green pepper, tomatoes, bay leaf, salt, pepper, and hot sauce. Let it simmer for another 30 minutes.

---

3. Saute the okra in the butter over the lowest heat for about 5 minutes, then add to the soup, and simmer just 10 minutes more.

4. Just before serving, stir in the cream and sprinkle just a touch of paprika on each serving.

Yield: 6 servings, each with 16 grams of carbohydrates and 5 grams of fiber, for a total of 11 grams of usable carbs and 49 grams of protein.

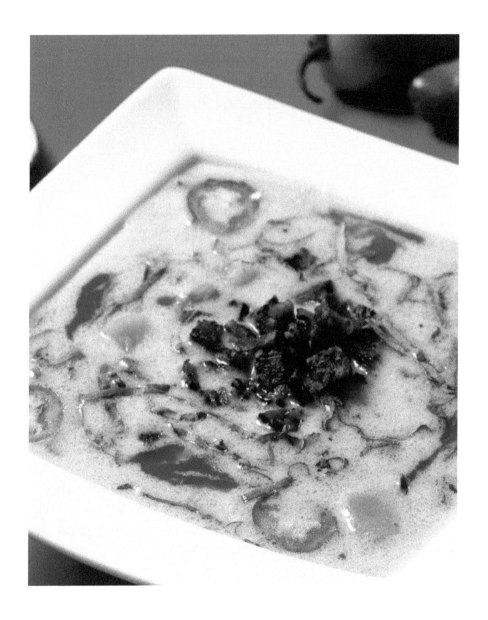

# Eggdrop Soup

Quick and easy, but filling, and it can practically save your life when you've got a cold. You don't have to use the guar, but it gives the broth the same rich quality that the cornstarch-thickened Chinese broths have.

1 quart chicken broth
1/4 teaspoon guar (optional)
1 tablespoon soy sauce
1 tablespoon rice vinegar
1/2 teaspoon grated fresh ginger
1 scallion, sliced
2 eggs

1. Put a cup or so of the chicken broth in your blender, turn it on Low, and add the guar (if using). Let it blend for a second, then put it in a large saucepan with the rest of the broth. (If you're not using the guar, just put the broth directly in a saucepan.)
2. Add the soy sauce, rice vinegar, ginger, and scallion. Heat over medium-high heat, and let it simmer for 5 minutes or so to let the flavors blend.
3. Beat your eggs in a glass measuring cup or small pitcher-something with a pouring lip. Use a fork to stir the surface of the soup in a slow circle and pour in about 1/4 of the eggs, stirring as they cook and turn into shreds (which will happen almost instantaneously). Repeat three more times, using up all the egg, then serve!

Yield: 3 biggish servings, or 4 to 5 small ones (but this recipe is easy to double). In 4 servings, each will have 2 grams of carbohydrates, a trace of fiber, and 8 grams of protein.

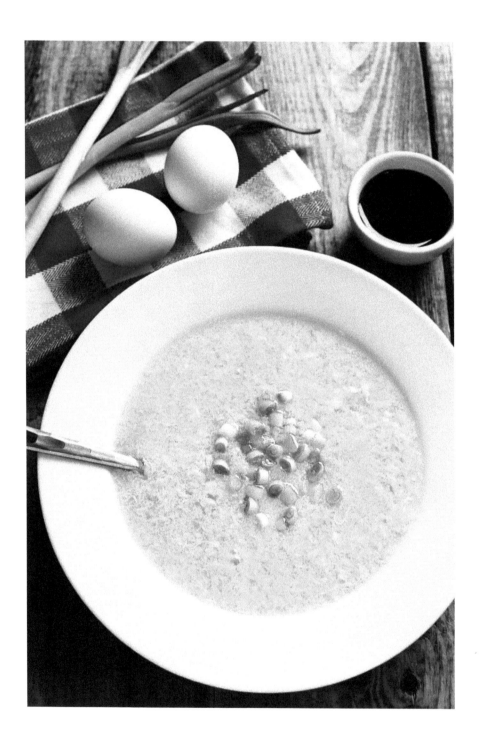

# *Stracciatella*

This is the Italian take on eggdrop soup, and it's delightful.

1 quart chicken broth
2 eggs
1/2 cup grated Parmesan cheese
1/2 teaspoon lemon juice
Pinch of nutmeg
1/2 teaspoon dried marjoram

1. Put 1/4 cup of the broth in a glass measuring cup or small pitcher. Pour the rest into a large saucepan over medium heat.
2. Add the eggs to the broth in the measuring cup, and beat with a fork. Then add the Parmesan, lemon juice, and nutmeg, and beat with a fork until well blended.
3. When the broth in the saucepan is simmering, stir it with a fork as you add small amounts of the egg and cheese mixture, until it's all stirred in.

Don't expect this to form long shreds like Chinese eggdrop soup; because of
the Parmesan, it makes small, fluffy particles, instead.

4. Add the marjoram, crushing it a bit between your fingers, and simmer the soup for another minute or so before serving.

---

Yield: 4 servings, each with 2 grams of carbohydrates,a trace of fiber, and 12 grams of protein.

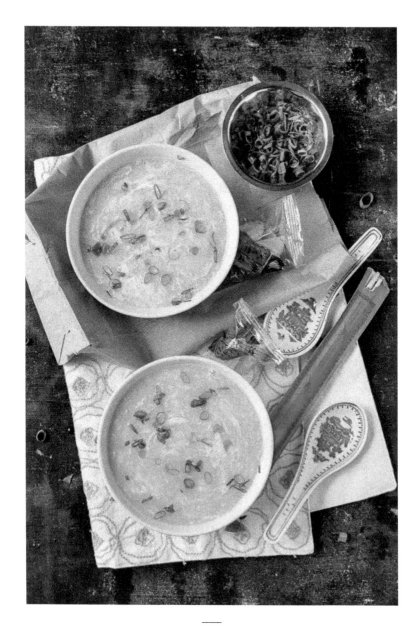

# *Manhattan Clam Chowder*

4 slices bacon, diced
1 large onion, chopped
2 ribs celery, diced
1 green pepper, chopped
2 1/2 cups diced white turnip
1 grated carrot
1 can (14 1/2 ounces) diced tomatoes
3 cups water
1 teaspoon dried thyme
4 cans (6 1/2 ounces each) minced clams, including
liquid
Tabasco
1 teaspoon salt or Vege-Sal
1 teaspoon pepper

1. In a large, heavy bottomed stock pot, start the bacon cooking. As the fat cooks out of it, add the onion, celery, and green pepper, and saute them in the bacon fat for 4 to 5 minutes.
2. Add the turnip, carrot, tomatoes, water, and thyme, and let the whole thing simmer for 30 minutes to 1 hour.
3. Add the clams, including the liquid, a dash of Tabasco, the salt or Vege-Sal, and pepper. Simmer for another 15 minutes, and serve.

Yield: 10 servings, each with 11 grams of carbohydrates and 1 gram of fiber, for a total of 10 grams of usable carbs and 21 grams of protein.

---

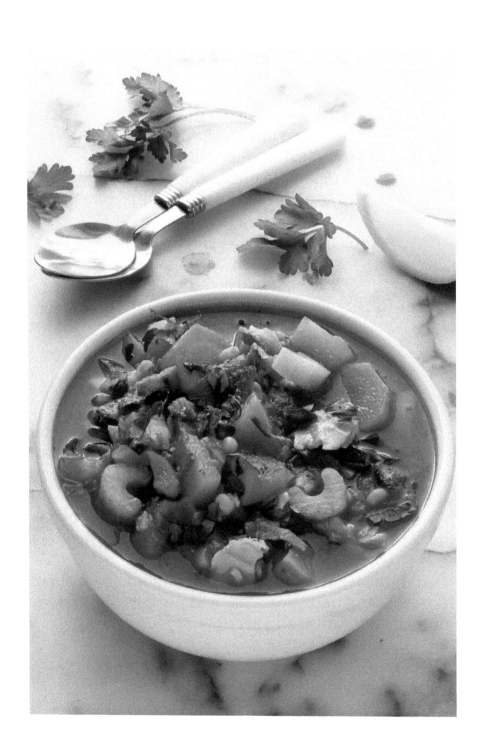

# Lo-Carb Clam Chowder

New England Clam Chowder fans will want to try this recipe from reader Tricia Hudgins.

8 pieces bacon
1/2 cup finely chopped onion
1/2 cup finely chopped celery
2 cans clams (6 1/2 ounces each), drained and with
the juice reserved
1 cup chicken broth
2 large turnips, peeled and chopped into small cubes
1/2 teaspoon pepper
1/2 teaspoon dried thyme
Salt
1 cup heavy cream

1. Fry the bacon and set it aside, reserving the bacon grease. Saute the onion and celery in 3 tablespoons of the bacon grease until they're soft.
2. Remove the onion and celery from the heat, and add the clam juice, chicken broth, turnips, pepper, thyme, and salt. Cover and cook over medium heat, stirring occasionally, until the turnips are soft (about 15 minutes).
3. Remove from the heat and stir in the heavy cream and clams. Crumble the bacon. and add it to the soup. Reheat over a low flame, and serve.

Yield: 4 servings, each with 13 grams of carbohydrates and 2 grams of fiber, for a

---

total of 11 grams of usable carbs and 31 grams of protein.

The sharp or bitter part of the turnip is the outside layer near the skin. Peel
your turnips with a paring knife, being careful to get all of the outer layer.

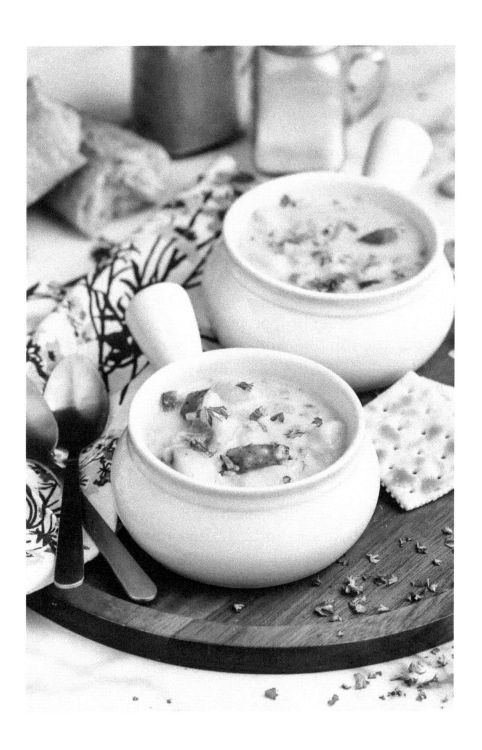

# Quick Green Chowder

1 package (10 ounces) frozen chopped spinach,
thawed
2 cans (6 1/2 ounces each) minced clams, including
the liquid
1 cup half-and-half
1 cup heavy cream
1 cup water
Salt and pepper

1. Put the spinach, clams, half-and-half, cream, and water in a blender or food processor, and puree.
2. Pour the mixture into a saucepan, and bring to a simmer (use very low heat, and don't boil!). Simmer for 5 minutes, and salt and pepper to taste.

~ If you prefer, you can puree everything but the clams, adding them later so they stay in chunks.

Yield: 4 servings, each with 12 grams of carbohydrates and 2 grams of fiber, for a total of 10 grams of usable carbs and 29 grams of protein.

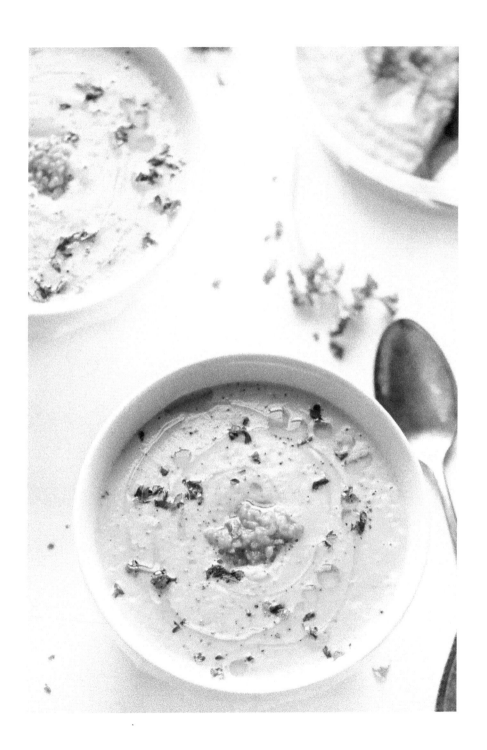

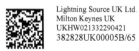

Lightning Source UK Ltd.
Milton Keynes UK
UKHW021332290421
382828UK00005B/65

9 781802 676167